TH

MET FLEX DIET

WORKBOOK

A COMPANION TO THE MET FLEX DIET PROGRAM

Ian K. Smith, M.D.

#1 *NY Times* Bestselling Author

The Ancient Nine

The Blackbird Papers

THE

MET FLEX DIET

WORKBOOK

A COMPANION TO THE MET FLEX DIET PROGRAM

Ian K. Smith, M.D.

#1 *NY Times* Bestselling Author

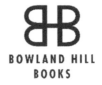

BOWLAND HILL
BOOKS

This book contains a guide to be used as a supplement to the MET FLEX DIET. This is not a diet, rather a companion to the diet program. If you know or suspect you have a health problem, it is recommended that you seek your physician's advice before embarking on any medical program or treatment. All efforts have been made to ensure the accuracy of the information contained in this book as of the date of publication. This publisher and the author disclaim liability for any medical outcomes that may occur as a result of applying the methods suggested in this book.

First published in the United States by Bowland Hill Books

www.DoctorIanSmith.com

Instagram: @doctoriansmith

Facebook: https://www.facebook.com/Dr.IanKSmith

Twitter: @DrIanSmith

TikTok: theofficialdrian

YouTube: @GetFitWithDrIan

ISBN: 9798378720156

FIRST EDITION: 2023

10 | 9 | 8 | 7 | 6 | 5 | 4 | 3 | 2 | 1

MET FLEX DIET Workbook

This is your workbook to chart your progress on your **MET FLEX DIET** journey. Knowing where you've been and where you are helps to better inform and give context to the vision of where you want and can go. This workbook is an extremely useful device that will allow you to take stock of your journey and help keep you accountable to yourself and the goals you've set out to achieve. Be honest, open, and reflective as you chart your journey, but equally important, always remain hopeful. One of the biggest catalysts to success is consistency. Remember, **CONSISTENCY LEADS TO PROGRESS LEADS TO SUCCESS!** This workbook is meant to be tight and considerate of your time. You only need 7 minutes a day to make it work for you. That is not a lot of time, but it's a great use of 420 seconds. It's essential that you make this a priority. You will learn so much about yourself and it will help you better embrace the process of transformation that you will be undergoing. This workbook is YOURS! It's a living, breathing record that you can reflect upon, review, and be inspired by as you move through this expedition. Continue to remind yourself, especially when things get tough or you might be disappointed, why you decided to begin making this change in your life in the first place. And no matter what, stay in the fight! Progress might not be as fast as you want, but slow progress will still get you down the road and where you want to go.

BELIEVE IN YOURSELF. WORK HARD. HAVE FUN!

Ian K. Smith, M.D.

MISSION STATEMENT (What you are trying to accomplish overall and why.)

_____

_____

_____

_____

_____

_____

_____

S.M.A.R.T. GOALS (Your goals should be Specific, Measurable, Achievable, Relevant, and Time bound. For example, don't just say, "I want to lose weight." Instead, say, "I want to lose 20 lbs. in 5 months.")

1._____

2._____

3._____

4._____

5._____

STRONG HABITS (Those habits you already possess that positively impact your mission/goals.)

1._____

2._____

3._____

4._____

5._____

WEAK HABITS (Those habits you need to change to fulfill or meet your mission/goals.)

1._____

2._____

3._____

4._____

5._____

GUIDING AFFIRMATION (A statement or series of statements that emotionally support and encourage you to stay positive and steadfast in the execution of your mission and pursuit of your goals. This statement can be as long or as short as you want, but you should read it at least once a day, and not just when things are difficult, but when they are good also.)

_____

_____

_____

_____

_____

_____

_____

_____

WEEK 1 PLANNER

Name 3 mini goals for this week as they relate to your larger, overall goals.

1._____

2._____

3._____

Identify your support. (Which person, persons, group, or activity will you engage for support.)

_____

FUN! FUN! FUN! (What you will do this week to have fun that has NOTHING to do with following the program, but also won't put you at odds with the program's guidelines or your mission/goals.)

1._____

2._____

3._____

4._____

5._____

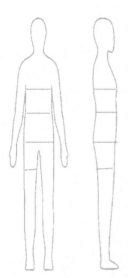

How to measure.

Chest-Stand and exhale so that your lungs are not full of air, then wrap the measuring tape just above the nipple line.

Waist-Stand and find the midway point between the top of your hip bone on the side of your body (iliac crest) and the bottom of your rib cage. This is typically the narrowest point at your waist.

Hips-Stand and measure the largest point of girth which is where your buttocks protrudes the most.

Thigh-Stand and measure just below your buttocks as this is typically the location of the largest girth. Measure both thighs.

Chest_____

Waist_____

Hips_____

Thighs
(L)_____

(R)_____

Weight (including number after decimal point)

Date
Taken_____

Weight_____

DAY 1

Daily Word (A single word that best describes your mood, psychological state, determination, or overall general feeling. You can use this word for as many days as it applies. Each day does not have to be a new word.)

_____

Daily Work (1-3 things you are going to work on today as it relates to your mission/goals.)

1._____

2._____

3._____

Daily Assessment (Complete this before going to bed.)

How did you do with regard to your daily work? (1-No effort; 2-Unsatisfactory; 3-Satisfactory; 4-Better than satisfactory; 5-Exceeded expectations)

_____

What prevented you from accomplishing your work today?

_____

_____

What was instrumental in helping you accomplish your work today?

_____

_____

Write a short, encouraging sentence to yourself for tomorrow.

_____

_____

DAY 2

Daily Word (A single word that best describes your mood, psychological state, determination, or overall general feeling. You can use this word for as many days as it applies. Each day does not have to be a new word.)

_____

Daily Work (1-3 things you are going to work on today as it relates to your mission/goals.)

1._____

2._____

3._____

Daily Assessment (Complete this before going to bed.)

How did you do with regard to your daily work? (1-No effort; 2-Unsatisfactory; 3-Satisfactory; 4-Better than satisfactory; 5-Exceeded expectations)

_____

What prevented you from accomplishing your work today?

_____

_____

What was instrumental in helping you accomplish your work today?

_____

_____

Write a short, encouraging sentence to yourself for tomorrow.

_____

_____

DAY 3

Daily Word (A single word that best describes your mood, psychological state, determination, or overall general feeling. You can use this word for as many days as it applies. Each day does not have to be a new word.)

_____

Daily Work (1-3 things you are going to work on today as it relates to your mission/goals.)

1._____

2._____

3._____

Daily Assessment (Complete this before going to bed.)

How did you do with regard to your daily work? (1-No effort; 2-Unsatisfactory; 3-Satisfactory; 4-Better than satisfactory; 5-Exceeded expectations)

_____

What prevented you from accomplishing your work today?

_____

What was instrumental in helping you accomplish your work today?

_____

Write a short, encouraging sentence to yourself for tomorrow.

_____

_____

DAY 4

Daily Word (A single word that best describes your mood, psychological state, determination, or overall general feeling. You can use this word for as many days as it applies. Each day does not have to be a new word.)

_____

Daily Work (1-3 things you are going to work on today as it relates to your mission/goals.)

1._____

2._____

3._____

Daily Assessment (Complete this before going to bed.)

How did you do with regard to your daily work? (1-No effort; 2-Unsatisfactory; 3-Satisfactory; 4-Better than satisfactory; 5-Exceeded expectations)

_____

What prevented you from accomplishing your work today?

_____

What was instrumental in helping you accomplish your work today?

_____

Write a short, encouraging sentence to yourself for tomorrow.

_____

_____

DAY 5

Daily Word (A single word that best describes your mood, psychological state, determination, or overall general feeling. You can use this word for as many days as it applies. Each day does not have to be a new word.)

_____

Daily Work (1-3 things you are going to work on today as it relates to your mission/goals.)

1._____

2._____

3._____

Daily Assessment (Complete this before going to bed.)

How did you do with regard to your daily work? (1-No effort; 2-Unsatisfactory; 3-Satisfactory; 4-Better than satisfactory; 5-Exceeded expectations)

_____

What prevented you from accomplishing your work today?

_____

What was instrumental in helping you accomplish your work today?

_____

Write a short, encouraging sentence to yourself for tomorrow.

_____

_____

DAY 6

Daily Word (A single word that best describes your mood, psychological state, determination, or overall general feeling. You can use this word for as many days as it applies. Each day does not have to be a new word.)

_____

Daily Work (1-3 things you are going to work on today as it relates to your mission/goals.)

1._____

2._____

3._____

Daily Assessment (Complete this before going to bed.)

How did you do with regard to your daily work? (1-No effort; 2-Unsatisfactory; 3-Satisfactory; 4-Better than satisfactory; 5-Exceeded expectations)

_____

What prevented you from accomplishing your work today?

_____

What was instrumental in helping you accomplish your work today?

_____

Write a short, encouraging sentence to yourself for tomorrow.

_____

_____

DAY 7

Daily Word (A single word that best describes your mood, psychological state, determination, or overall general feeling. You can use this word for as many days as it applies. Each day does not have to be a new word.)

_____

Daily Work (1-3 things you are going to work on today as it relates to your mission/goals.)

1._____

2._____

3._____

Daily Assessment (Complete this before going to bed.)

How did you do with regard to your daily work? (1-No effort; 2-Unsatisfactory; 3-Satisfactory; 4-Better than satisfactory; 5-Exceeded expectations)

_____

What prevented you from accomplishing your work today?

_____

What was instrumental in helping you accomplish your work today?

_____

Write a short, encouraging sentence to yourself for tomorrow.

_____

_____

WEEK 1

PHYSICAL ASSESSMENT

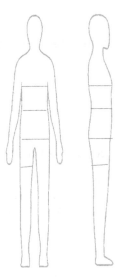

How to measure.

Chest-Stand and exhale so that your lungs are not full of air, then wrap the measuring tape just above the nipple line.

Waist-Stand and find the midway point between the top of your hip bone on the side of your body (iliac crest) and the bottom of your rib cage. This is typically the narrowest point at your waist.

Hips-Stand and measure the largest point of girth which is where your buttocks protrudes the most.

Thigh-Stand and measure just below your buttocks-typically the location of the largest girth. Measure both thighs.

Chest_____

Waist_____

Hips_____

Thighs
(L)_____

(R)_____

Weight (including number after decimal point)

Date
Taken_____

Weight_____

END OF WEEK INVENTORY ASSESSMENT

It's always important to take stock of what has occurred in your journey to give you perspective and context for moving forward. Take the time and be honest in your assessment.

Which mini goals did you reach?

1._____

2._____

3._____

4._____

5._____

Which mini goals did you not reach?

1._____

2._____

3._____

4._____

5._____

What are your overall feelings about how you did this past week/how you will do next week?

This week

_____

_____

Next week

_____

_____

WEEK 2 PLANNER

Name 3 mini goals for this week as they relate to your larger, overall goals.

1._____

2._____

3._____

Identify your support. (Which person, persons, group, or activity will you engage for support.)

_____

_____

FUN! FUN! FUN! (What you will do this week to have fun that has NOTHING to do with following the program, but also won't put you at odds with the program's guidelines or your mission/goals.)

1._____

2._____

3._____

4._____

5._____

DAY 8

Daily Word (A single word that best describes your mood, psychological state, determination, or overall general feeling. You can use this word for as many days as it applies. Each day does not have to be a new word.)

_____

Daily Work (1-3 things you are going to work on today as it relates to your mission/goals.)

1._____

2._____

3._____

Daily Assessment (Complete this before going to bed.)

How did you do with regard to your daily work? (1-No effort; 2-Unsatisfactory; 3-Satisfactory; 4-Better than satisfactory; 5-Exceeded expectations)

_____

What prevented you from accomplishing your work today?

_____

What was instrumental in helping you accomplish your work today?

_____

Write a short, encouraging sentence to yourself for tomorrow.

_____

_____

DAY 9

Daily Word (A single word that best describes your mood, psychological state, determination, or overall general feeling. You can use this word for as many days as it applies. Each day does not have to be a new word.)

_____

Daily Work (1-3 things you are going to work on today as it relates to your mission/goals.)

1._____

2._____

3._____

Daily Assessment (Complete this before going to bed.)

How did you do with regard to your daily work? (1-No effort; 2-Unsatisfactory; 3-Satisfactory; 4-Better than satisfactory; 5-Exceeded expectations)

_____

What prevented you from accomplishing your work today?

_____

What was instrumental in helping you accomplish your work today?

_____

Write a short, encouraging sentence to yourself for tomorrow.

_____

_____

DAY 10

Daily Word (A single word that best describes your mood, psychological state, determination, or overall general feeling. You can use this word for as many days as it applies. Each day does not have to be a new word.)

_____

Daily Work (1-3 things you are going to work on today as it relates to your mission/goals.)

1._____

2._____

3._____

Daily Assessment (Complete this before going to bed.)

How did you do with regard to your daily work? (1-No effort; 2-Unsatisfactory; 3-Satisfactory; 4-Better than satisfactory; 5-Exceeded expectations)

_____

What prevented you from accomplishing your work today?

_____

What was instrumental in helping you accomplish your work today?

_____

Write a short, encouraging sentence to yourself for tomorrow.

_____

_____

DAY 11

Daily Word (A single word that best describes your mood, psychological state, determination, or overall general feeling. You can use this word for as many days as it applies. Each day does not have to be a new word.)

_____

Daily Work (1-3 things you are going to work on today as it relates to your mission/goals.)

1._____

2._____

3._____

Daily Assessment (Complete this before going to bed.)

How did you do with regard to your daily work? (1-No effort; 2-Unsatisfactory; 3-Satisfactory; 4-Better than satisfactory; 5-Exceeded expectations)

_____

What prevented you from accomplishing your work today?

_____

What was instrumental in helping you accomplish your work today?

_____

Write a short, encouraging sentence to yourself for tomorrow.

_____

_____

DAY 12

Daily Word (A single word that best describes your mood, psychological state, determination, or overall general feeling. You can use this word for as many days as it applies. Each day does not have to be a new word.)

_____

Daily Work (1-3 things you are going to work on today as it relates to your mission/goals.)

1._____

2._____

3._____

Daily Assessment (Complete this before going to bed.)

How did you do with regard to your daily work? (1-No effort; 2-Unsatisfactory; 3-Satisfactory; 4-Better than satisfactory; 5-Exceeded expectations)

_____

What prevented you from accomplishing your work today?

_____

What was instrumental in helping you accomplish your work today?

_____

Write a short, encouraging sentence to yourself for tomorrow.

_____

_____

DAY 13

Daily Word (A single word that best describes your mood, psychological state, determination, or overall general feeling. You can use this word for as many days as it applies. Each day does not have to be a new word.)

_____

Daily Work (1-3 things you are going to work on today as it relates to your mission/goals.)

1._____

2._____

3._____

Daily Assessment (Complete this before going to bed.)

How did you do with regard to your daily work? (1-No effort; 2-Unsatisfactory; 3-Satisfactory; 4-Better than satisfactory; 5-Exceeded expectations)

_____

What prevented you from accomplishing your work today?

_____

What was instrumental in helping you accomplish your work today?

_____

Write a short, encouraging sentence to yourself for tomorrow.

_____

_____

DAY 14

Daily Word (A single word that best describes your mood, psychological state, determination, or overall general feeling. You can use this word for as many days as it applies. Each day does not have to be a new word.)

_____

Daily Work (1-3 things you are going to work on today as it relates to your mission/goals.)

1._____

2._____

3._____

Daily Assessment (Complete this before going to bed.)

How did you do with regard to your daily work? (1-No effort; 2-Unsatisfactory; 3-Satisfactory; 4-Better than satisfactory; 5-Exceeded expectations)

_____

What prevented you from accomplishing your work today?

_____

What was instrumental in helping you accomplish your work today?

_____

Write a short, encouraging sentence to yourself for tomorrow.

_____

_____

WEEK 2

PHYSICAL ASSESSMENT

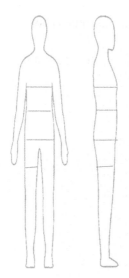

How to measure.

Chest-Stand and exhale so that your lungs are not full of air, then wrap the measuring tape just above the nipple line.

Waist-Stand and find the midway point between the top of your hip bone on the side of your body (iliac crest) and the bottom of your rib cage. This is typically the narrowest point at your waist.

Hips-Stand and measure the largest point of girth which is where your buttocks protrudes the most.

Thigh-Stand and measure just below your buttocks-typically the location of the largest girth. Measure both thighs.

Chest_____

Waist_____

Hips_____

Thighs
(L)_____

(R)_____

Weight (including number after decimal point)

Date
Taken_____

Weight_____

END OF WEEK INVENTORY ASSESSMENT

It's always important to take stock of what has occurred in your journey to give you perspective and context for moving forward. Take the time and be honest in your assessment.

Which mini goals did you reach?

1._____

2._____

3._____

4._____

5._____

Which mini goals did you not reach?

1._____

2._____

3._____

4._____

5._____

What are your overall feelings about how you did this

past week/how you will do next week?

This week

_____

_____

Next week

_____

_____

WEEK 3 PLANNER

Name 3 mini goals for this week as they relate to your larger, overall goals.

1._____

2._____

3._____

Identify your support. (Which person, persons, group, or activity will you engage for support.)

_____

_____

FUN! FUN! FUN! (What you will do this week to have fun that has NOTHING to do with following the program, but also won't put you at odds with the program's guidelines or your mission/goals.)

1._____

2._____

3._____

4._____

5._____

DAY 15

Daily Word (A single word that best describes your mood, psychological state, determination, or overall general feeling. You can use this word for as many days as it applies. Each day does not have to be a new word.)

_____

Daily Work (1-3 things you are going to work on today as it relates to your mission/goals.)

1._____

2._____

3._____

Daily Assessment (Complete this before going to bed.)

How did you do with regard to your daily work? (1-No effort; 2-Unsatisfactory; 3-Satisfactory; 4-Better than satisfactory; 5-Exceeded expectations)

_____

What prevented you from accomplishing your work today?

_____

What was instrumental in helping you accomplish your work today?

_____

Write a short, encouraging sentence to yourself for tomorrow.

_____

_____

DAY 16

Daily Word (A single word that best describes your mood, psychological state, determination, or overall general feeling. You can use this word for as many days as it applies. Each day does not have to be a new word.)

_____

Daily Work (1-3 things you are going to work on today as it relates to your mission/goals.)

1._____

2._____

3._____

Daily Assessment (Complete this before going to bed.)

How did you do with regard to your daily work? (1-No effort; 2-Unsatisfactory; 3-Satisfactory; 4-Better than satisfactory; 5-Exceeded expectations)

_____

What prevented you from accomplishing your work today?

_____

What was instrumental in helping you accomplish your work today?

_____

Write a short, encouraging sentence to yourself for tomorrow.

_____

_____

What was instrumental in helping you accomplish your work today?

_____

_____

Write a short, encouraging sentence to yourself for tomorrow.

_____

_____

DAY 17

Daily Word (A single word that best describes your mood, psychological state, determination, or overall general feeling. You can use this word for as many days as it applies. Each day does not have to be a new word.)

_____

Daily Work (1-3 things you are going to work on today as it relates to your mission/goals.)

1._____

2._____

3._____

Daily Assessment (Complete this before going to bed.)

How did you do with regard to your daily work? (1-No effort; 2-Unsatisfactory; 3-Satisfactory; 4-Better than satisfactory; 5-Exceeded expectations)

_____

What prevented you from accomplishing your work today?

_____

What was instrumental in helping you accomplish your work today?

_____

Write a short, encouraging sentence to yourself for tomorrow.

_____

_____

DAY 18

Daily Word (A single word that best describes your mood, psychological state, determination, or overall general feeling. You can use this word for as many days as it applies. Each day does not have to be a new word.)

_____

Daily Work (1-3 things you are going to work on today as it relates to your mission/goals.)

1._____

2._____

3._____

Daily Assessment (Complete this before going to bed.)

How did you do with regard to your daily work? (1-No effort; 2-Unsatisfactory; 3-Satisfactory; 4-Better than satisfactory; 5-Exceeded expectations)

_____

What prevented you from accomplishing your work today?

_____

What was instrumental in helping you accomplish your work today?

_____

Write a short, encouraging sentence to yourself for tomorrow.

_____

_____

DAY 19

Daily Word (A single word that best describes your mood, psychological state, determination, or overall general feeling. You can use this word for as many days as it applies. Each day does not have to be a new word.)

_____

Daily Work (1-3 things you are going to work on today as it relates to your mission/goals.)

1._____

2._____

3._____

Daily Assessment (Complete this before going to bed.)

How did you do with regard to your daily work? (1-No effort; 2-Unsatisfactory; 3-Satisfactory; 4-Better than satisfactory; 5-Exceeded expectations)

_____

What prevented you from accomplishing your work today?

_____

What was instrumental in helping you accomplish your work today?

_____

Write a short, encouraging sentence to yourself for tomorrow.

_____

_____

DAY 20

Daily Word (A single word that best describes your mood, psychological state, determination, or overall general feeling. You can use this word for as many days as it applies. Each day does not have to be a new word.)

_____

Daily Work (1-3 things you are going to work on today as it relates to your mission/goals.)

1._____

2._____

3._____

Daily Assessment (Complete this before going to bed.)

How did you do with regard to your daily work? (1-No effort; 2-Unsatisfactory; 3-Satisfactory; 4-Better than satisfactory; 5-Exceeded expectations)

_____

What prevented you from accomplishing your work today?

_____

What was instrumental in helping you accomplish your work today?

_____

Write a short, encouraging sentence to yourself for tomorrow.

_____

_____

DAY 21

Daily Word (A single word that best describes your mood, psychological state, determination, or overall general feeling. You can use this word for as many days as it applies. Each day does not have to be a new word.)

_____

Daily Work (1-3 things you are going to work on today as it relates to your mission/goals.)

1._____

2._____

3._____

Daily Assessment (Complete this before going to bed.)

How did you do with regard to your daily work? (1-No effort; 2-Unsatisfactory; 3-Satisfactory; 4-Better than satisfactory; 5-Exceeded expectations)

_____

What prevented you from accomplishing your work today?

_____

What was instrumental in helping you accomplish your work today?

_____

Write a short, encouraging sentence to yourself for tomorrow.

_____

_____

WEEK 3

PHYSICAL ASSESSMENT

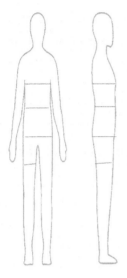

How to measure.

Chest-Stand and exhale so that your lungs are not full of air, then wrap the measuring tape just above the nipple line.

Waist-Stand and find the midway point between the top of your hip bone on the side of your body (iliac crest) and the bottom of your rib cage. This is typically the narrowest point at your waist.

Hips-Stand and measure the largest point of girth which is where your buttocks protrudes the most.

Thigh-Stand and measure just below your buttocks-typically the location of the largest girth. Measure both thighs.

Chest_____

Waist_____

Hips_____

Thighs
(L)_____

(R)_____

Weight (including number after decimal point)

Date
Taken_____

Weight_____

END OF WEEK INVENTORY ASSESSMENT

It's always important to take stock of what has occurred in your journey to give you perspective and context for moving forward. Take the time and be honest in your assessment.

Which mini goals did you reach?

1._____

2._____

3._____

4._____

5._____

Which mini goals did you not reach?

1._____

2._____

3._____

4._____

5._____

What are your overall feelings about how you did this past week/how you will do next week?

This week

_____

_____

Next week

_____

_____

WEEK 4 PLANNER

Name 3 mini goals for this week as they relate to your larger, overall goals.

1. _____

2. _____

3. _____

Identify your support. (Which person, persons, group, or activity will you engage for support.)

_____

_____

FUN! FUN! FUN! (What you will do this week to have fun that has NOTHING to do with following the program, but also won't put you at odds with the program's guidelines or your mission/goals.)

1._____

2._____

3._____

4._____

5._____

DAY 22

Daily Word (A single word that best describes your mood, psychological state, determination, or overall general feeling. You can use this word for as many days as it applies. Each day does not have to be a new word.)

_____

Daily Work (1-3 things you are going to work on today as it relates to your mission/goals.)

1._____

2._____

3._____

Daily Assessment (Complete this before going to bed.)

How did you do with regard to your daily work? (1-No effort; 2-Unsatisfactory; 3-Satisfactory; 4-Better than satisfactory; 5-Exceeded expectations)

_____

What prevented you from accomplishing your work today?

_____

What was instrumental in helping you accomplish your work today?

_____

Write a short, encouraging sentence to yourself for tomorrow.

_____

_____

DAY 23

Daily Word (A single word that best describes your mood, psychological state, determination, or overall general feeling. You can use this word for as many days as it applies. Each day does not have to be a new word.)

_____

Daily Work (1-3 things you are going to work on today as it relates to your mission/goals.)

1._____

2._____

3._____

Daily Assessment (Complete this before going to bed.)

How did you do with regard to your daily work? (1-No effort; 2-Unsatisfactory; 3-Satisfactory; 4-Better than satisfactory; 5-Exceeded expectations)

_____

What prevented you from accomplishing your work today?

_____

What was instrumental in helping you accomplish your work today?

_____

Write a short, encouraging sentence to yourself for tomorrow.

_____

_____

DAY 24

Daily Word (A single word that best describes your mood, psychological state, determination, or overall general feeling. You can use this word for as many days as it applies. Each day does not have to be a new word.)

_____

Daily Work (1-3 things you are going to work on today as it relates to your mission/goals.)

1._____

2._____

3._____

Daily Assessment (Complete this before going to bed.)

How did you do with regard to your daily work? (1-No effort; 2-Unsatisfactory; 3-Satisfactory; 4-Better than satisfactory; 5-Exceeded expectations)

_____

What prevented you from accomplishing your work today?

_____

What was instrumental in helping you accomplish your work today?

_____

Write a short, encouraging sentence to yourself for tomorrow.

_____

_____

DAY 25

Daily Word (A single word that best describes your mood, psychological state, determination, or overall general feeling. You can use this word for as many days as it applies. Each day does not have to be a new word.)

_____

Daily Work (1-3 things you are going to work on today as it relates to your mission/goals.)

1._____

2._____

3._____

Daily Assessment (Complete this before going to bed.)

How did you do with regard to your daily work? (1-No effort; 2-Unsatisfactory; 3-Satisfactory; 4-Better than satisfactory; 5-Exceeded expectations)

_____

What prevented you from accomplishing your work today?

_____

What was instrumental in helping you accomplish your work today?

_____

Write a short, encouraging sentence to yourself for tomorrow.

_____

_____

DAY 26

Daily Word (A single word that best describes your mood, psychological state, determination, or overall general feeling. You can use this word for as many days as it applies. Each day does not have to be a new word.)

_____

Daily Work (1-3 things you are going to work on today as it relates to your mission/goals.)

1._____

2._____

3._____

Daily Assessment (Complete this before going to bed.)

How did you do with regard to your daily work? (1-No effort; 2-Unsatisfactory; 3-Satisfactory; 4-Better than satisfactory; 5-Exceeded expectations)

_____

What prevented you from accomplishing your work today?

_____

What was instrumental in helping you accomplish your work today?

_____

Write a short, encouraging sentence to yourself for tomorrow.

_____

_____

DAY 27

Daily Word (A single word that best describes your mood, psychological state, determination, or overall general feeling. You can use this word for as many days as it applies. Each day does not have to be a new word.)

_____

Daily Work (1-3 things you are going to work on today as it relates to your mission/goals.)

1._____

2._____

3._____

Daily Assessment (Complete this before going to bed.)

How did you do with regard to your daily work? (1-No effort; 2-Unsatisfactory; 3-Satisfactory; 4-Better than satisfactory; 5-Exceeded expectations)

_____

What prevented you from accomplishing your work today?

_____

What was instrumental in helping you accomplish your work today?

_____

Write a short, encouraging sentence to yourself for tomorrow.

_____

_____

DAY 28

Daily Word (A single word that best describes your mood, psychological state, determination, or overall general feeling. You can use this word for as many days as it applies. Each day does not have to be a new word.)

_____

Daily Work (1-3 things you are going to work on today as it relates to your mission/goals.)

1._____

2._____

3._____

Daily Assessment (Complete this before going to bed.)

How did you do with regard to your daily work? (1-No effort; 2-Unsatisfactory; 3-Satisfactory; 4-Better than satisfactory; 5-Exceeded expectations)

_____

What prevented you from accomplishing your work today?

_____

What was instrumental in helping you accomplish your work today?

_____

Write a short, encouraging sentence to yourself for tomorrow.

_____

_____

WEEK 4

PHYSICAL ASSESSMENT

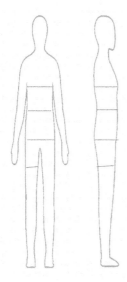

How to measure.

Chest-Stand and exhale so that your lungs are not full of air, then wrap the measuring tape just above the nipple line.

Waist-Stand and find the midway point between the top of your hip bone on the side of your body (iliac crest) and the bottom of your rib cage. This is typically the narrowest point at your waist.

Hips-Stand and measure the largest point of girth which is where your buttocks protrudes the most.

Thigh-Stand and measure just below your buttocks-typically the location of the largest girth. Measure both thighs.

Chest_____

Waist_____

Hips_____

Thighs (L)_____

(R)_____

Weight (including number after decimal point)

Date Taken_____

Weight_____

END OF WEEK INVENTORY ASSESSMENT

It's always important to take stock of what has occurred in your journey to give you perspective and context for moving forward. Take the time and be honest in your assessment.

Which mini goals did you reach?

1._____

2._____

3._____

4._____

5._____

Which mini goals did you not reach?

1._____

2._____

3._____

4._____

5._____

What are your overall feelings about how you did this past week/how you will do next week?

This week

_____

_____

Next week

_____

_____

WEEK 5 PLANNER

Name 3 mini goals for this week as they relate to your larger, overall goals.

1._____

2._____

3._____

Identify your support. (Which person, persons, group, or activity will you engage for support.)

_____

_____

FUN! FUN! FUN! (What you will do this week to have fun that has NOTHING to do with following the program, but also won't put you at odds with the program's guidelines or your mission/goals.)

1._____

2._____

3._____

4._____

5._____

DAY 29

Daily Word (A single word that best describes your mood, psychological state, determination, or overall general feeling. You can use this word for as many days as it applies. Each day does not have to be a new word.)

_____

Daily Work (1-3 things you are going to work on today as it relates to your mission/goals.)

1._____

2._____

3._____

Daily Assessment (Complete this before going to bed.)

How did you do with regard to your daily work? (1-No effort; 2-Unsatisfactory; 3-Satisfactory; 4-Better than satisfactory; 5-Exceeded expectations)

_____

What prevented you from accomplishing your work today?

_____

What was instrumental in helping you accomplish your work today?

_____

Write a short, encouraging sentence to yourself for tomorrow.

_____

_____

DAY 30

Daily Word (A single word that best describes your mood, psychological state, determination, or overall general feeling. You can use this word for as many days as it applies. Each day does not have to be a new word.)

_____

Daily Work (1-3 things you are going to work on today as it relates to your mission/goals.)

1._____

2._____

3._____

Daily Assessment (Complete this before going to bed.)

How did you do with regard to your daily work? (1-No effort; 2-Unsatisfactory; 3-Satisfactory; 4-Better than satisfactory; 5-Exceeded expectations)

_____

What prevented you from accomplishing your work today?

_____

What was instrumental in helping you accomplish your work today?

_____

Write a short, encouraging sentence to yourself for tomorrow.

_____

_____

DAY 31

Daily Word (A single word that best describes your mood, psychological state, determination, or overall general feeling. You can use this word for as many days as it applies. Each day does not have to be a new word.)

_____

Daily Work (1-3 things you are going to work on today as it relates to your mission/goals.)

1._____

2._____

3._____

Daily Assessment (Complete this before going to bed.)

How did you do with regard to your daily work? (1-No effort; 2-Unsatisfactory; 3-Satisfactory; 4-Better than satisfactory; 5-Exceeded expectations)

_____

What prevented you from accomplishing your work today?

_____

What was instrumental in helping you accomplish your work today?

_____

Write a short, encouraging sentence to yourself for tomorrow.

_____
_____

DAY 32

Daily Word (A single word that best describes your mood, psychological state, determination, or overall general feeling. You can use this word for as many days as it applies. Each day does not have to be a new word.)

_____

Daily Work (1-3 things you are going to work on today as it relates to your mission/goals.)

1._____

2._____

3._____

Daily Assessment (Complete this before going to bed.)

How did you do with regard to your daily work? (1-No effort; 2-Unsatisfactory; 3-Satisfactory; 4-Better than satisfactory; 5-Exceeded expectations)

_____

What prevented you from accomplishing your work today?

_____

What was instrumental in helping you accomplish your work today?

_____

Write a short, encouraging sentence to yourself for tomorrow.

_____

_____

DAY 33

Daily Word (A single word that best describes your mood, psychological state, determination, or overall general feeling. You can use this word for as many days as it applies. Each day does not have to be a new word.)

_____

Daily Work (1-3 things you are going to work on today as it relates to your mission/goals.)

1._____

2._____

3._____

Daily Assessment (Complete this before going to bed.)

How did you do with regard to your daily work? (1-No effort; 2-Unsatisfactory; 3-Satisfactory; 4-Better than satisfactory; 5-Exceeded expectations)

_____

What prevented you from accomplishing your work today?

_____

What was instrumental in helping you accomplish your work today?

_____

Write a short, encouraging sentence to yourself for tomorrow.

_____

_____

DAY 34

Daily Word (A single word that best describes your mood, psychological state, determination, or overall general feeling. You can use this word for as many days as it applies. Each day does not have to be a new word.)

_____

Daily Work (1-3 things you are going to work on today as it relates to your mission/goals.)

1._____

2._____

3._____

Daily Assessment (Complete this before going to bed.)

How did you do with regard to your daily work? (1-No effort; 2-Unsatisfactory; 3-Satisfactory; 4-Better than satisfactory; 5-Exceeded expectations)

_____

What prevented you from accomplishing your work today?

_____

What was instrumental in helping you accomplish your work today?

_____

Write a short, encouraging sentence to yourself for tomorrow.

_____

_____

DAY 35

Daily Word (A single word that best describes your mood, psychological state, determination, or overall general feeling. You can use this word for as many days as it applies. Each day does not have to be a new word.)

_____

Daily Work (1-3 things you are going to work on today as it relates to your mission/goals.)

1._____

2._____

3._____

Daily Assessment (Complete this before going to bed.)

How did you do with regard to your daily work? (1-No effort; 2-Unsatisfactory; 3-Satisfactory; 4-Better than satisfactory; 5-Exceeded expectations)

_____

What prevented you from accomplishing your work today?

_____

What was instrumental in helping you accomplish your work today?

_____

Write a short, encouraging sentence to yourself for tomorrow.

_____

_____

WEEK 5

PHYSICAL ASSESSMENT

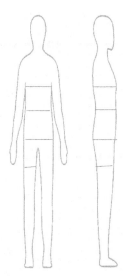

How to measure.

Chest-Stand and exhale so that your lungs are not full of air, then wrap the measuring tape just above the nipple line.

Waist-Stand and find the midway point between the top of your hip bone on the side of your body (iliac crest) and the bottom of your rib cage. This is typically the narrowest point at your waist.

Hips-Stand and measure the largest point of girth which is where your buttocks protrudes the most.

Thigh-Stand and measure just below your buttocks-typically the location of the largest girth. Measure both thighs.

Chest_____

Waist_____

Hips_____

Thighs
(L)_____

(R)_____

Weight (including number after decimal point)

Date
Taken_____

Weight_____

END OF WEEK INVENTORY ASSESSMENT

It's always important to take stock of what has occurred in your journey to give you perspective and context for moving forward. Take the time and be honest in your assessment.

Which mini goals did you reach?

1._____

2._____

3._____

4._____

5._____

Which mini goals did you not reach?

1._____

2._____

3._____

4._____

5._____

What are your overall feelings about how you did this past week/how you will do next week?

This week

_____

_____

Next week

_____

_____

WEEK 6 PLANNER

Name 3 mini goals for this week as they relate to your larger, overall goals.

1._____

2._____

3._____

Identify your support. (Which person, persons, group, or activity will you engage for support.)

_____

_____

FUN! FUN! FUN! (What you will do this week to have fun that has NOTHING to do with following the program, but also won't put you at odds with the program's guidelines or your mission/goals.)

1._____

2._____

3._____

4._____

5._____

DAY 36

Daily Word (A single word that best describes your mood, psychological state, determination, or overall general feeling. You can use this word for as many days as it applies. Each day does not have to be a new word.)

_____

Daily Work (1-3 things you are going to work on today as it relates to your mission/goals.)

1._____

2._____

3._____

Daily Assessment (Complete this before going to bed.)

How did you do with regard to your daily work? (1-No effort; 2-Unsatisfactory; 3-Satisfactory; 4-Better than satisfactory; 5-Exceeded expectations)

_____

What prevented you from accomplishing your work today?

_____

What was instrumental in helping you accomplish your work today?

_____

Write a short, encouraging sentence to yourself for tomorrow.

_____

_____

DAY 37

Daily Word (A single word that best describes your mood, psychological state, determination, or overall general feeling. You can use this word for as many days as it applies. Each day does not have to be a new word.)

_____

Daily Work (1-3 things you are going to work on today as it relates to your mission/goals.)

1._____

2._____

3._____

Daily Assessment (Complete this before going to bed.)

How did you do with regard to your daily work? (1-No effort; 2-Unsatisfactory; 3-Satisfactory; 4-Better than satisfactory; 5-Exceeded expectations)

_____

What prevented you from accomplishing your work today?

_____

What was instrumental in helping you accomplish your work today?

_____

Write a short, encouraging sentence to yourself for tomorrow.

_____

_____

DAY 38

Daily Word (A single word that best describes your mood, psychological state, determination, or overall general feeling. You can use this word for as many days as it applies. Each day does not have to be a new word.)

_____

Daily Work (1-3 things you are going to work on today as it relates to your mission/goals.)

1._____

2._____

3._____

Daily Assessment (Complete this before going to bed.)

How did you do with regard to your daily work? (1-No effort; 2-Unsatisfactory; 3-Satisfactory; 4-Better than satisfactory; 5-Exceeded expectations)

_____

What prevented you from accomplishing your work today?

_____

What was instrumental in helping you accomplish your work today?

_____

Write a short, encouraging sentence to yourself for tomorrow.

_____

_____

DAY 39

Daily Word (A single word that best describes your mood, psychological state, determination, or overall general feeling. You can use this word for as many days as it applies. Each day does not have to be a new word.)

_____

Daily Work (1-3 things you are going to work on today as it relates to your mission/goals.)

1._____

2._____

3._____

Daily Assessment (Complete this before going to bed.)

How did you do with regard to your daily work? (1-No effort; 2-Unsatisfactory; 3-Satisfactory; 4-Better than satisfactory; 5-Exceeded expectations)

_____

What prevented you from accomplishing your work today?

_____

What was instrumental in helping you accomplish your work today?

_____

Write a short, encouraging sentence to yourself for tomorrow.

_____

_____

DAY 40

Daily Word (A single word that best describes your mood, psychological state, determination, or overall general feeling. You can use this word for as many days as it applies. Each day does not have to be a new word.)

_____

Daily Work (1-3 things you are going to work on today as it relates to your mission/goals.)

1._____

2._____

3._____

Daily Assessment (Complete this before going to bed.)

How did you do with regard to your daily work? (1-No effort; 2-Unsatisfactory; 3-Satisfactory; 4-Better than satisfactory; 5-Exceeded expectations)

_____

What prevented you from accomplishing your work today?

_____

What was instrumental in helping you accomplish your work today?

_____

Write a short, encouraging sentence to yourself for tomorrow.

_____

_____

DAY 41

Daily Word (A single word that best describes your mood, psychological state, determination, or overall general feeling. You can use this word for as many days as it applies. Each day does not have to be a new word.)

_____

Daily Work (1-3 things you are going to work on today as it relates to your mission/goals.)

1._____

2._____

3._____

Daily Assessment (Complete this before going to bed.)

How did you do with regard to your daily work? (1-No effort; 2-Unsatisfactory; 3-Satisfactory; 4-Better than satisfactory; 5-Exceeded expectations)

_____

What prevented you from accomplishing your work today?

_____

What was instrumental in helping you accomplish your work today?

_____

Write a short, encouraging sentence to yourself for tomorrow.

_____

_____

DAY 42

Daily Word (A single word that best describes your mood, psychological state, determination, or overall general feeling. You can use this word for as many days as it applies. Each day does not have to be a new word.)

_____

Daily Work (1-3 things you are going to work on today as it relates to your mission/goals.)

1._____

2._____

3._____

Daily Assessment (Complete this before going to bed.)

How did you do with regard to your daily work? (1-No effort; 2-Unsatisfactory; 3-Satisfactory; 4-Better than satisfactory; 5-Exceeded expectations)

_____

What prevented you from accomplishing your work today?

_____

What was instrumental in helping you accomplish your work today?

_____

Write a short, encouraging sentence to yourself for tomorrow.

_____

_____

WEEK 6

PHYSICAL ASSESSMENT

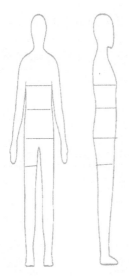

How to measure.

Chest-Stand and exhale so that your lungs are not full of air, then wrap the measuring tape just above the nipple line.

Waist-Stand and find the midway point between the top of your hip bone on the side of your body (iliac crest) and the bottom of your rib cage. This is typically the narrowest point at your waist.

Hips-Stand and measure the largest point of girth which is where your buttocks protrudes the most.

Thigh-Stand and measure just below your buttocks-typically the location of the largest girth. Measure both thighs.

Chest_____

Waist_____

Hips_____

Thighs
(L)_____

(R)_____

Weight (including number after decimal point)

Date
Taken_____

Weight_____

END OF WEEK INVENTORY ASSESSMENT

It's always important to take stock of what has occurred in your journey to give you perspective and context for moving forward. Take the time and be honest in your assessment.

Which mini goals did you reach?

1._____

2._____

3._____

4._____

5._____

Which mini goals did you not reach?

1._____

2._____

3._____

4._____

5._____

What are your overall feelings about how you did this past week/how you will do next week?

This week

_____

_____

Next week

_____

_____

Congratulations on completing this phase of the journey! You've been resilient and persistent, and hopefully you've worked hard to make great progress towards completing your mission and reaching some of your goals. The previous pages that you've filled in now serve as a testimony to what you can and need to do to achieve success. All that you've written the past six weeks now becomes a critical trove of your own personal research, a historical record that is full of insight and answers and inspiration to continue moving forward as you transform. Come back to it often to learn more about yourself and what you're capable of accomplishing.

It's important not to have the perspective that just because you've completed these six weeks, the journey is over. Honestly, the journey is never really over, rather it just takes different turns and sometimes different meanings and purposes. But that's the beauty of life and our desire to accomplish a mission. In many respects, you are not the same person you were six weeks ago and six weeks from now, you might be different in other aspects. Life is a constant evolution. It's a process of attempting and learning and modifying and adjusting. Be confident as you continue your expedition. Be kind to yourself knowing that no one is perfect, and we all will have our fair share of failures and successes. Both comprise the true texture of life, a gift that in even its saddest and darkest moments remains one to be treasured and respected. Life is short. Challenge yourself. Enjoy yourself. Love yourself. Travel well, my friend, and live for the most. You deserve nothing less!

Best,

Dr. Ian

Follow me on social media:

www.DoctorIanSmith.com

Instagram: @doctoriansmith

Facebook: https://www.facebook.com/Dr.IanKSmith

Twitter: @DrIanSmith

TikTok: theofficialdrian

YouTube: @GetFitWithDrIan

NOTES

Made in the USA
Las Vegas, NV
17 April 2023

70710403R00085